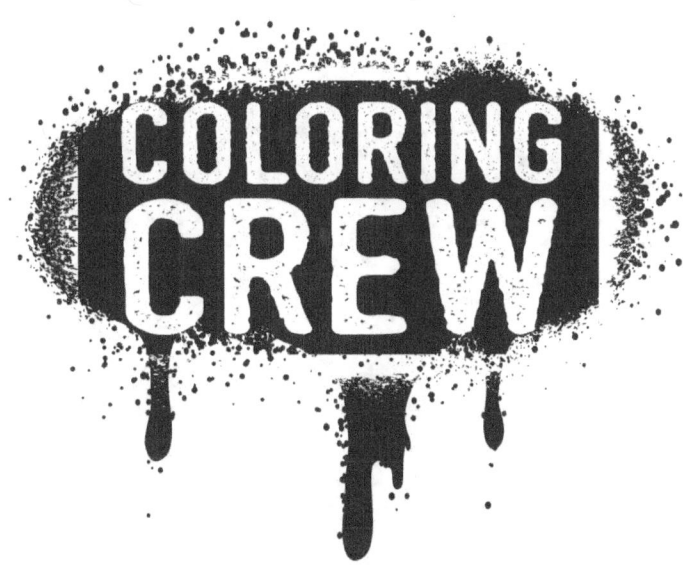

# IT'S OFFICIAL!
# YOU HAVE PROBLEMS!

BUT DON'T WORRY NOW YOU HAVE AN OUTLET FOR YOUR ANGER

INSIDE THIS BOOK YOU WILL FIND 20 MANDALAS FOR YOU TO SIT BACK AND COLOR

EACH ONE CONTAINS A PROBLEM THAT YOU SHOULD DEFINITELY BE ABLE TO RELATE TO!

## HAPPY COLORING

Copyright © 2018 Coloring Crew.
All rights reserved.
ISBN-13: 978-1985386648
ISBN-10: 198538664X

COLORING CREW

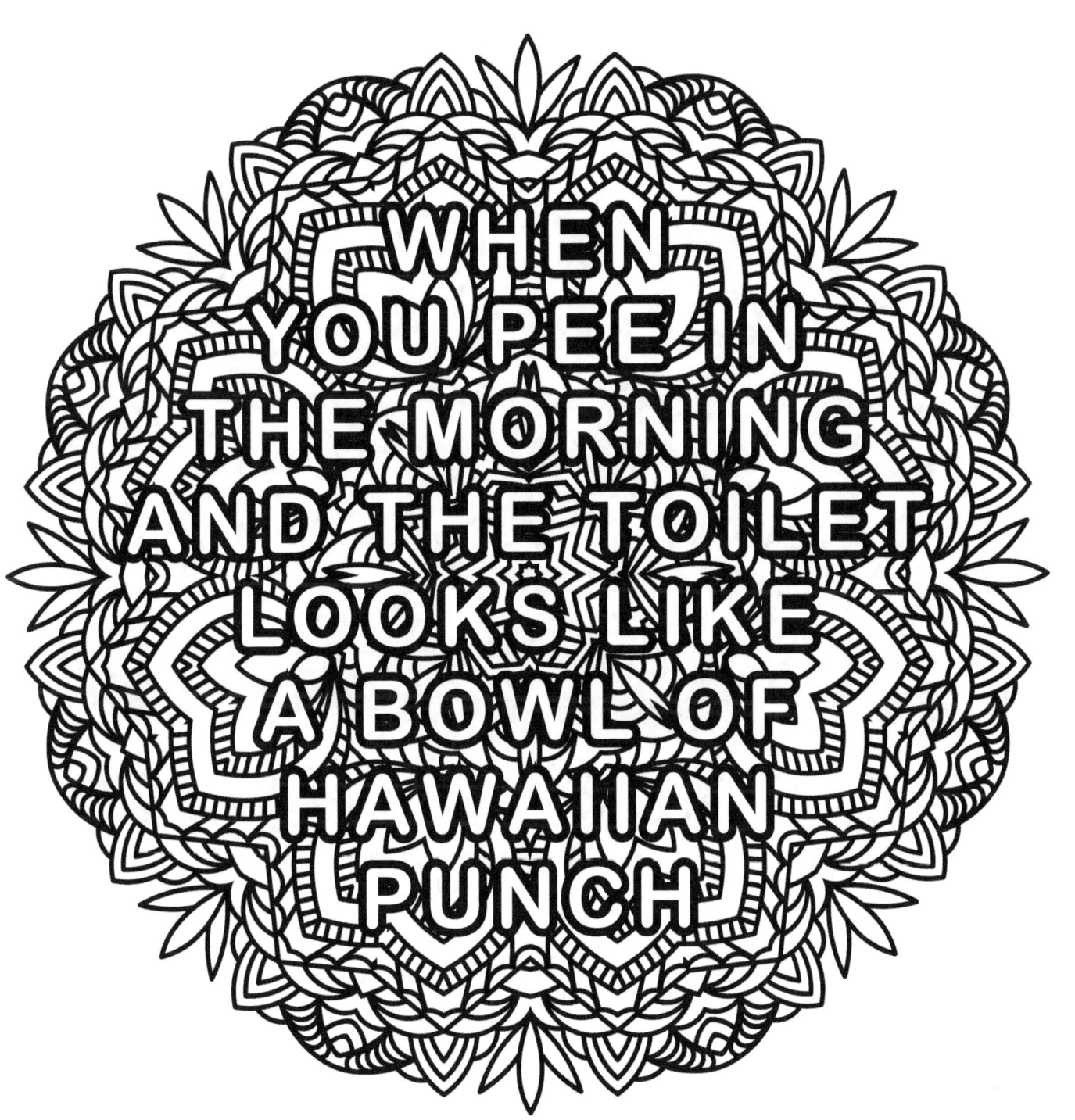

COLORING CREW

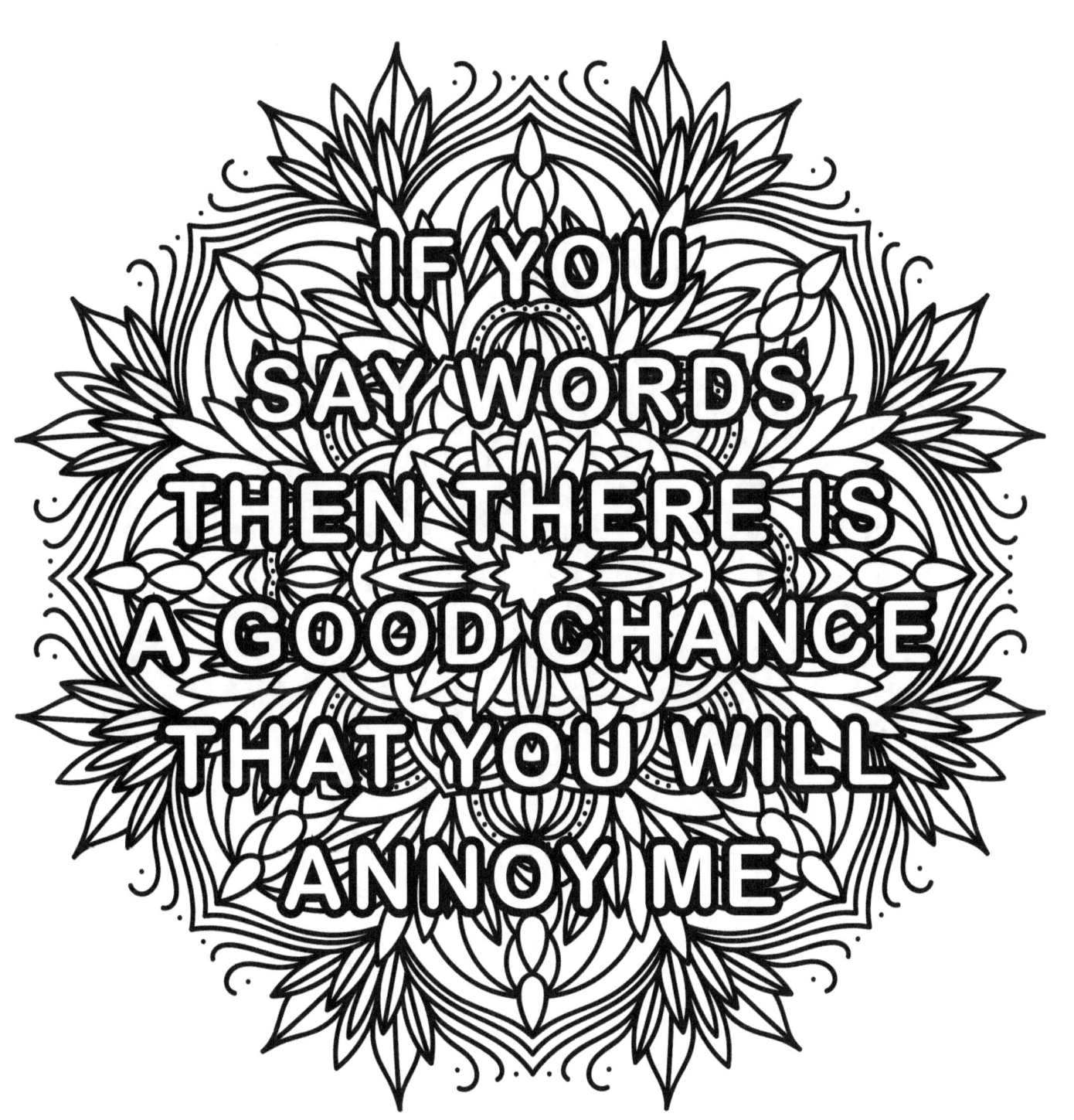

# COLORING CREW

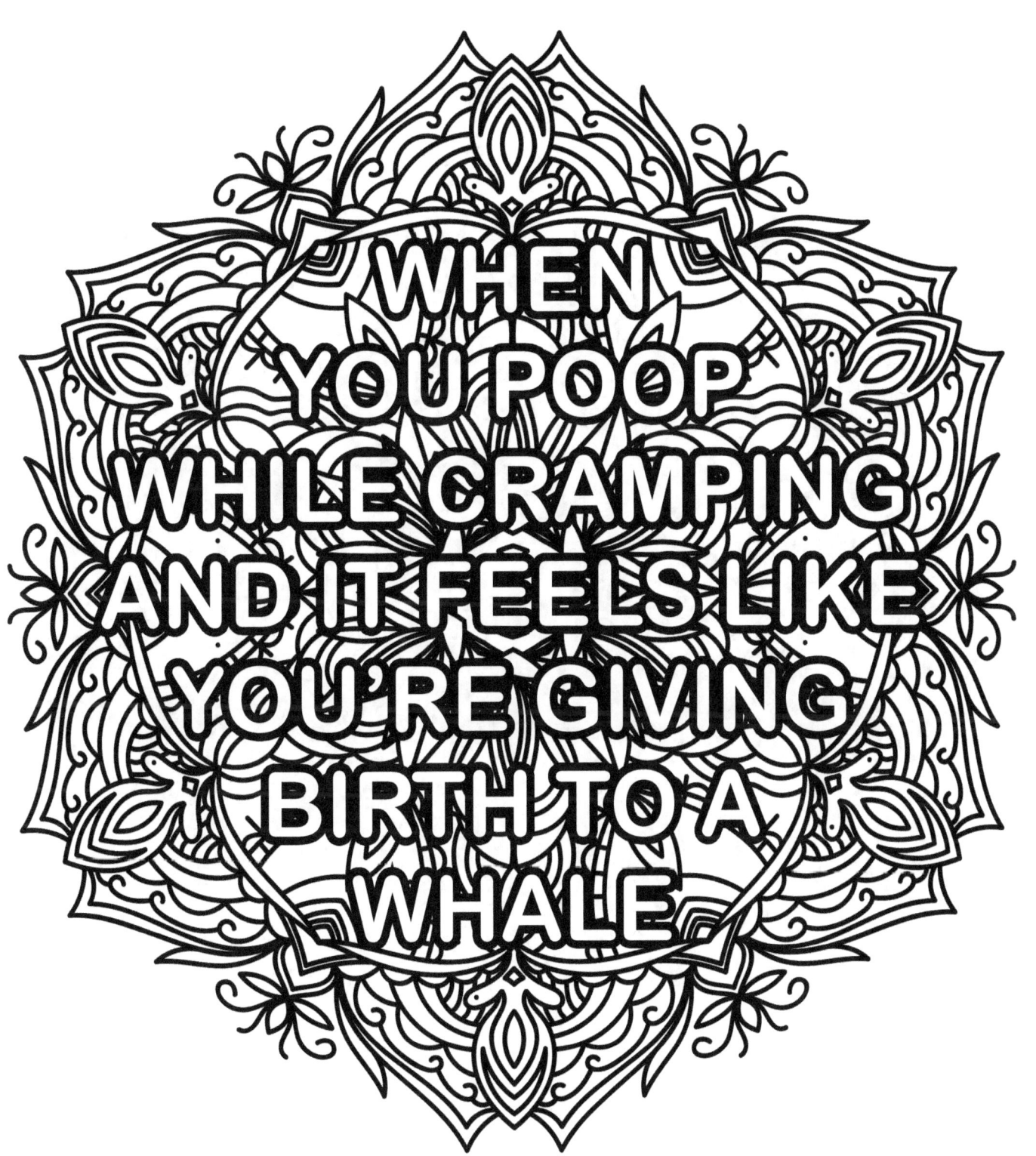

COLORING CREW

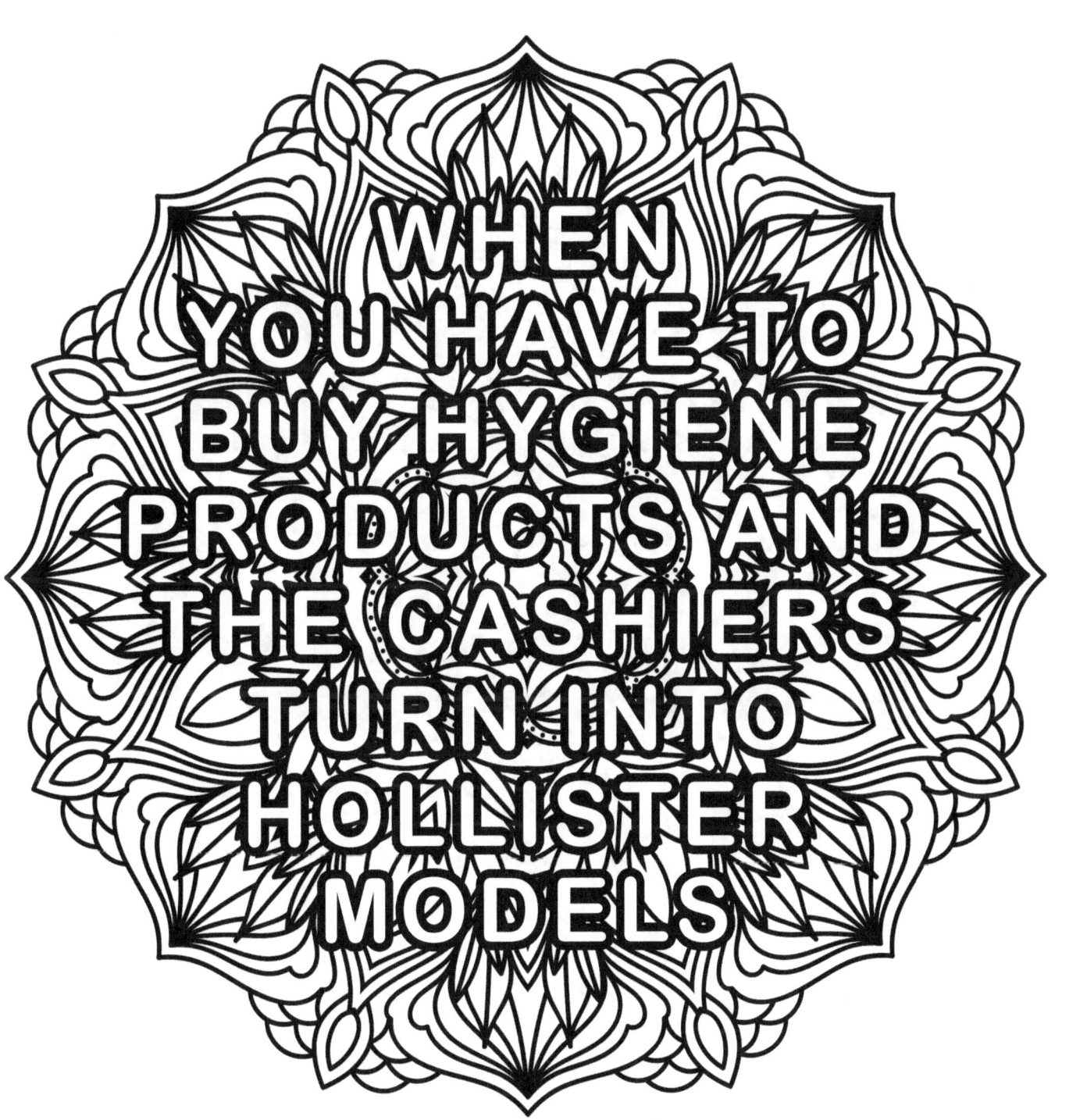

COLORING CREW

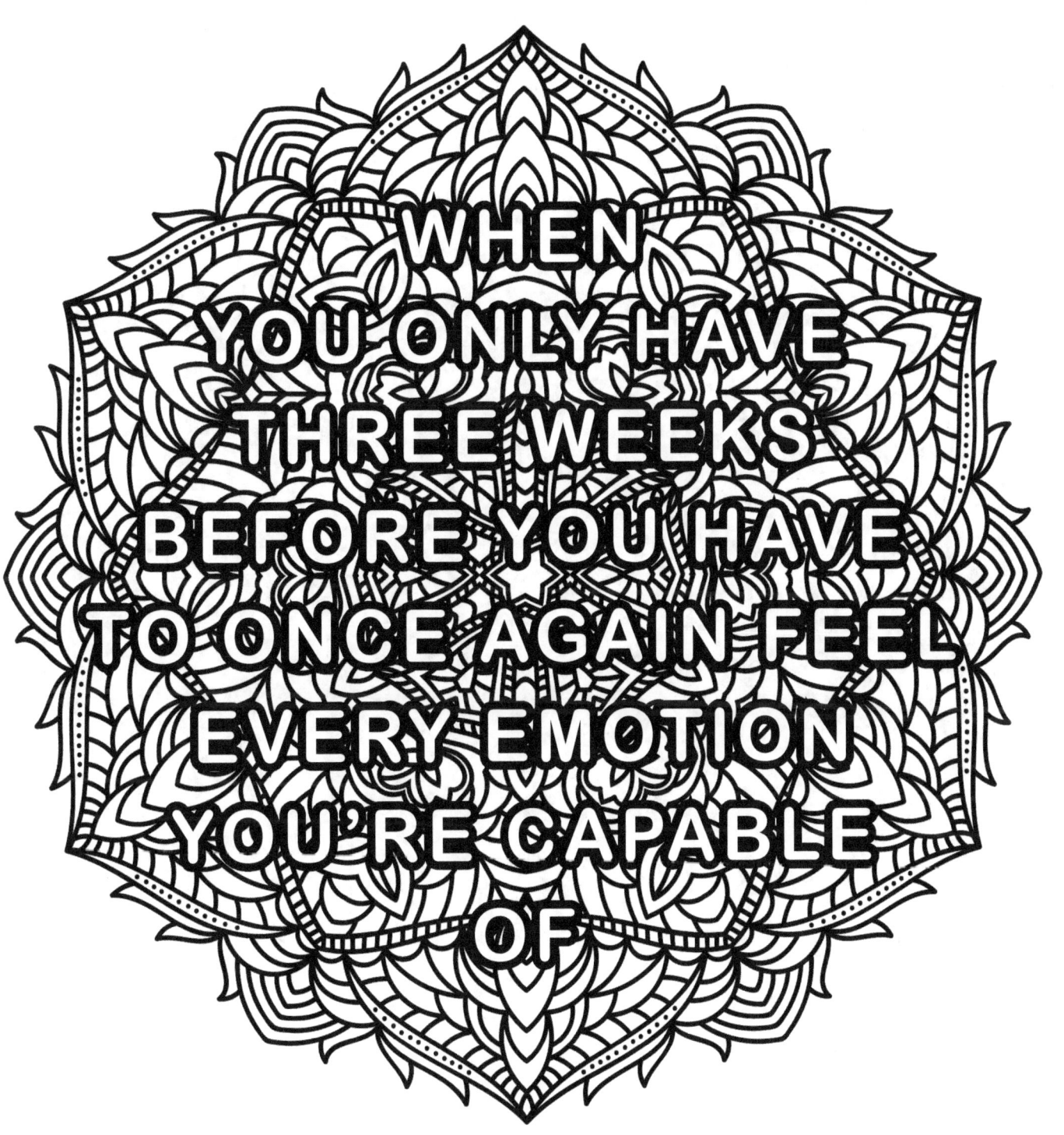

COLORING CREW

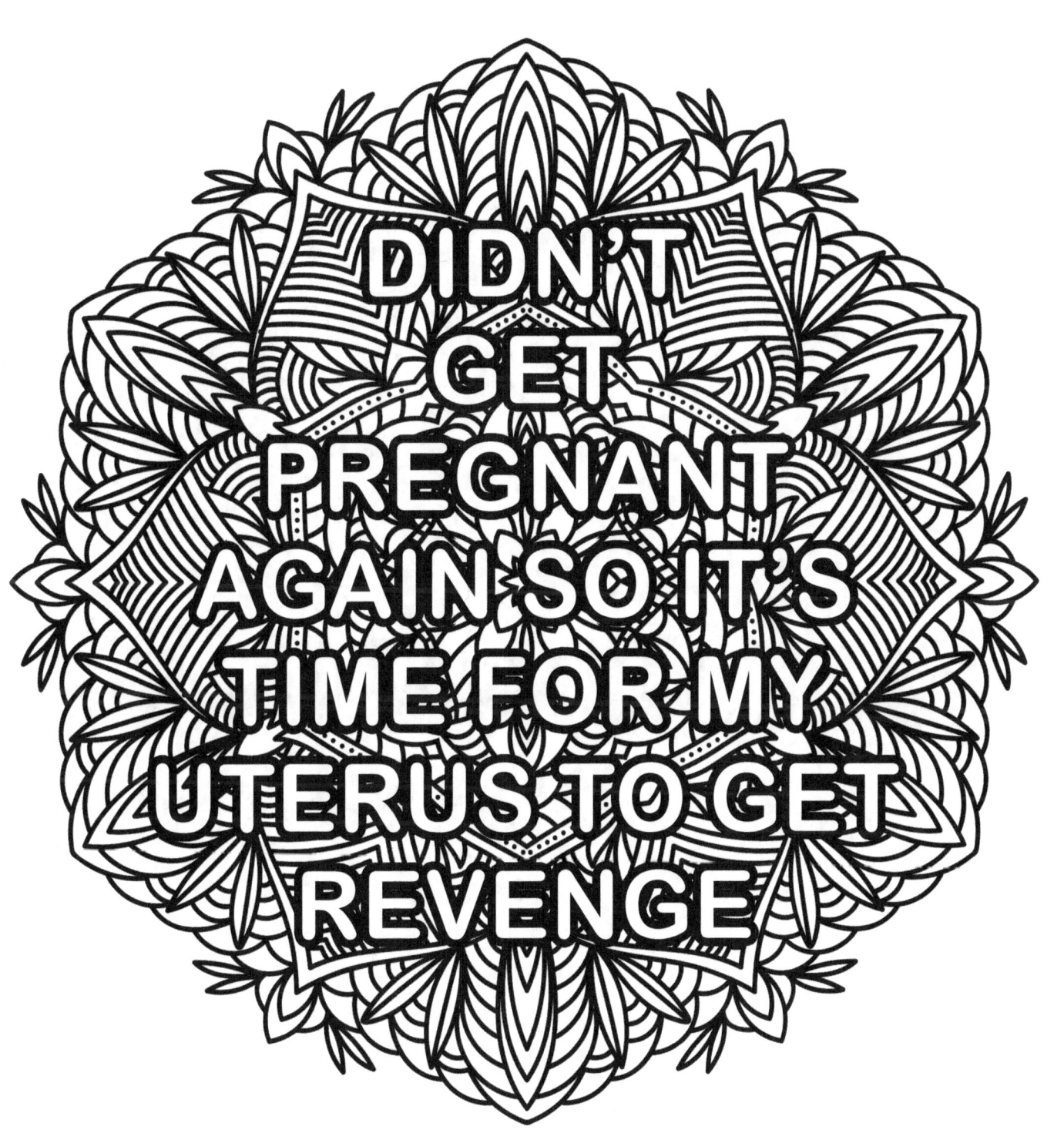

# COLORING CREW

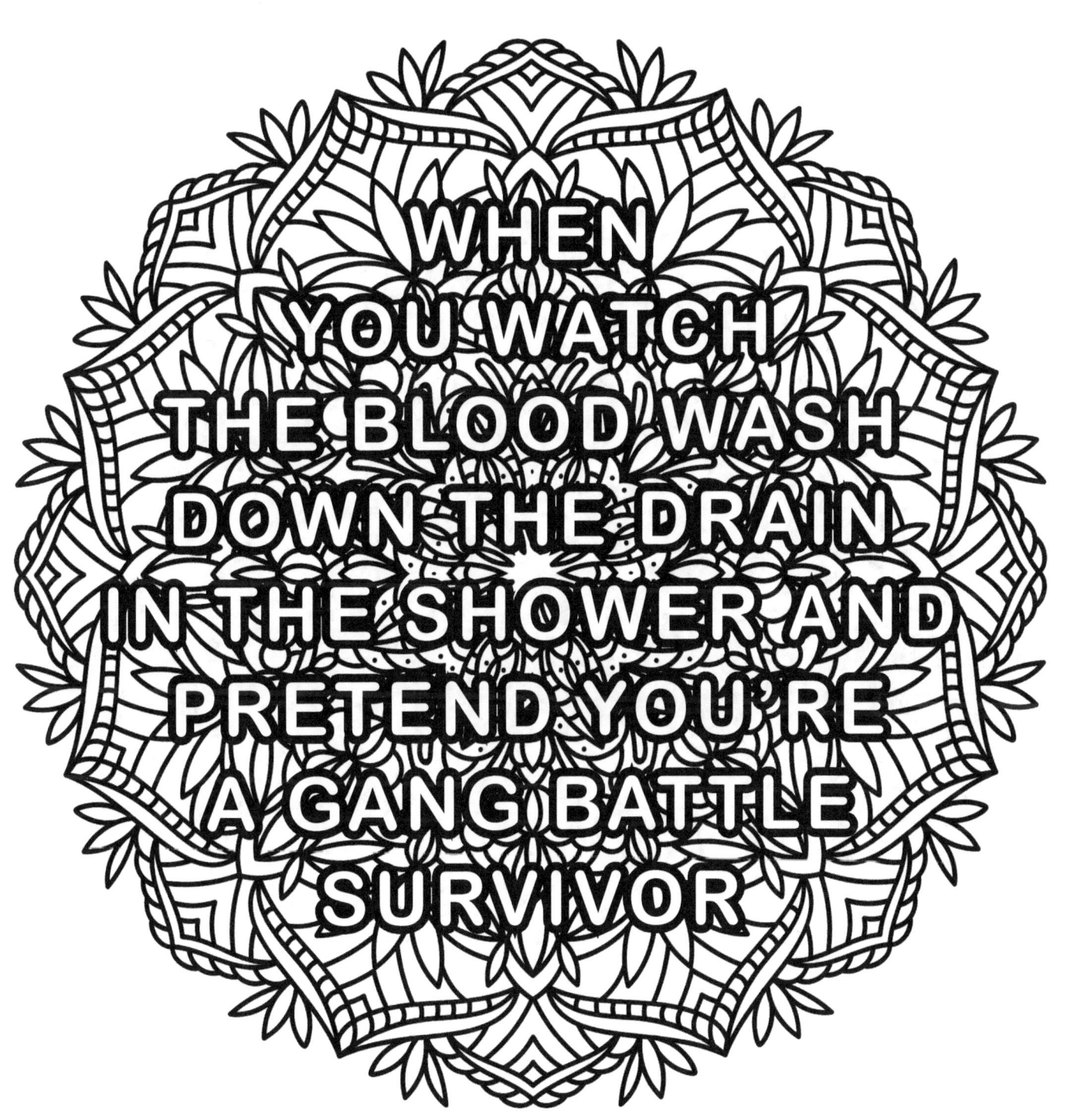

# COLORING CREW

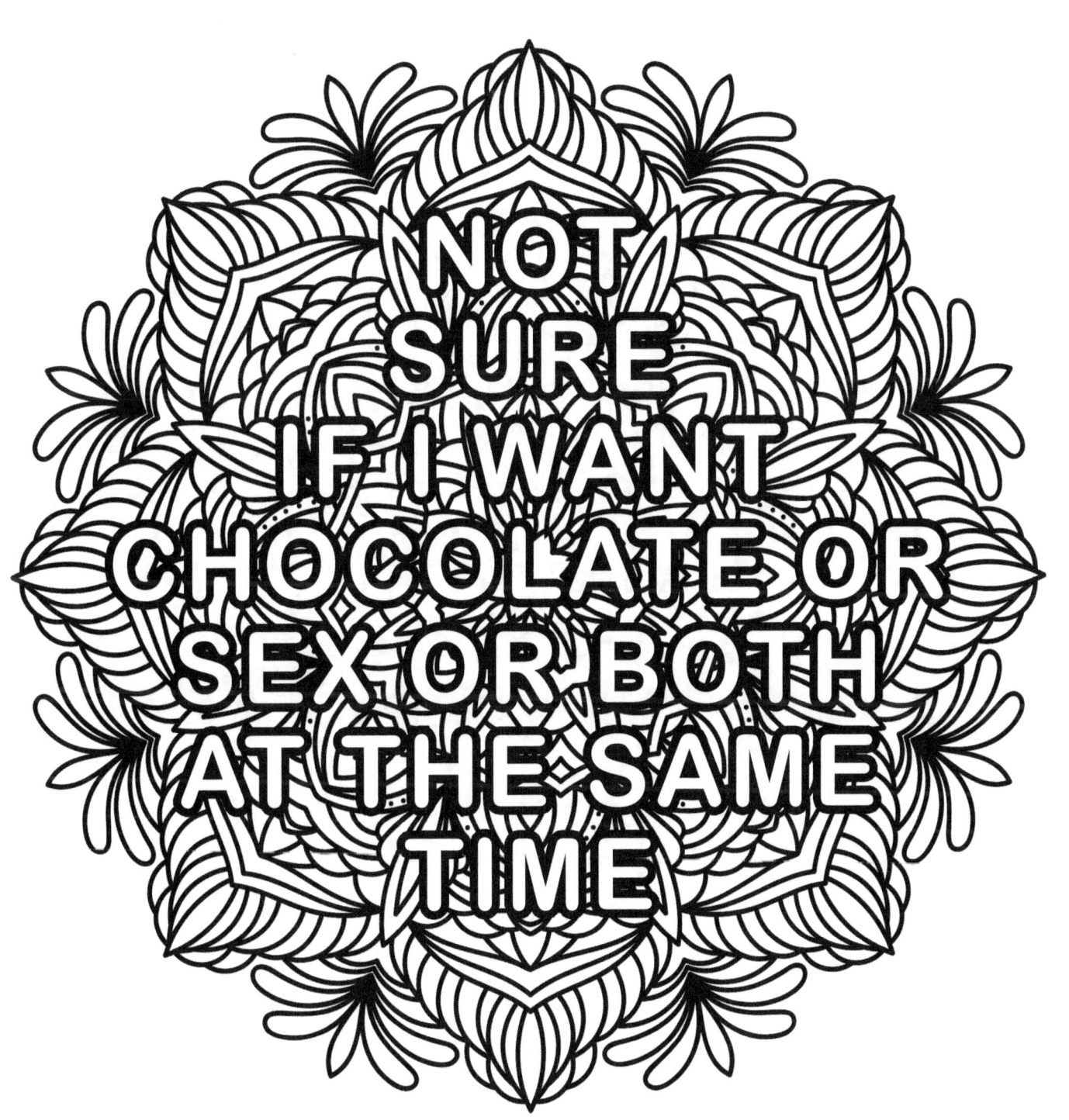

COLORING CREW

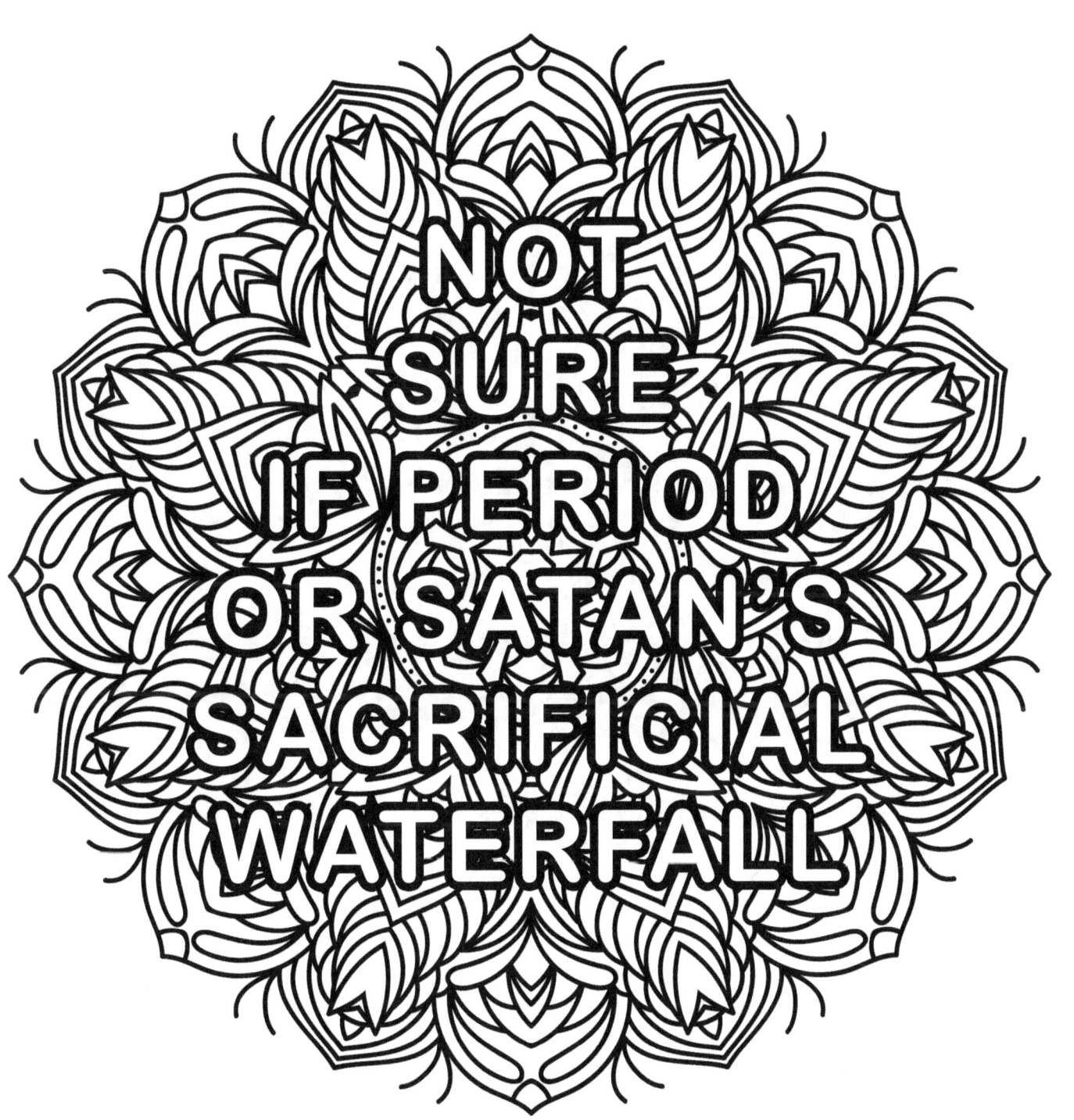

# COLORING CREW

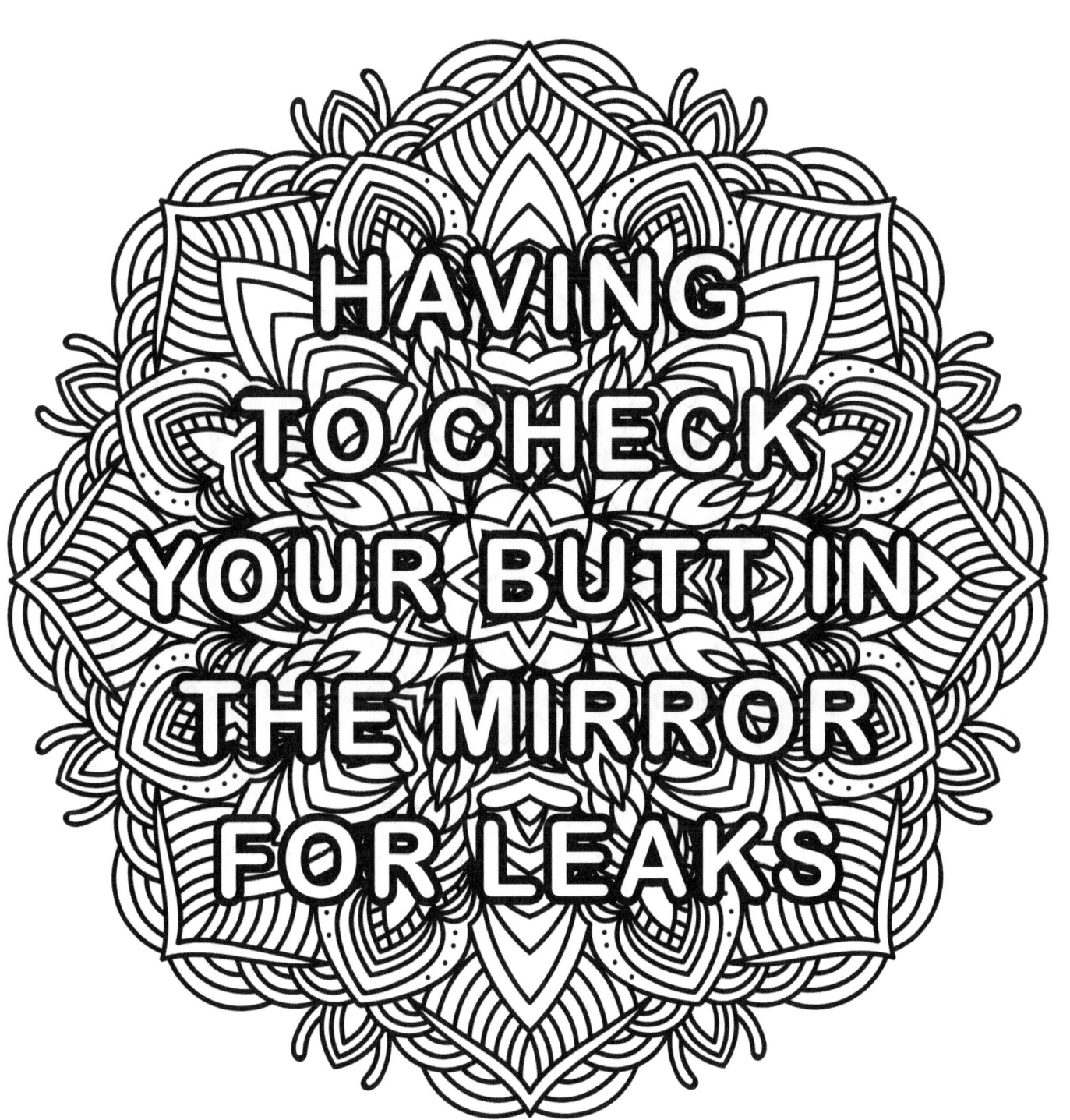

# COLORING CREW

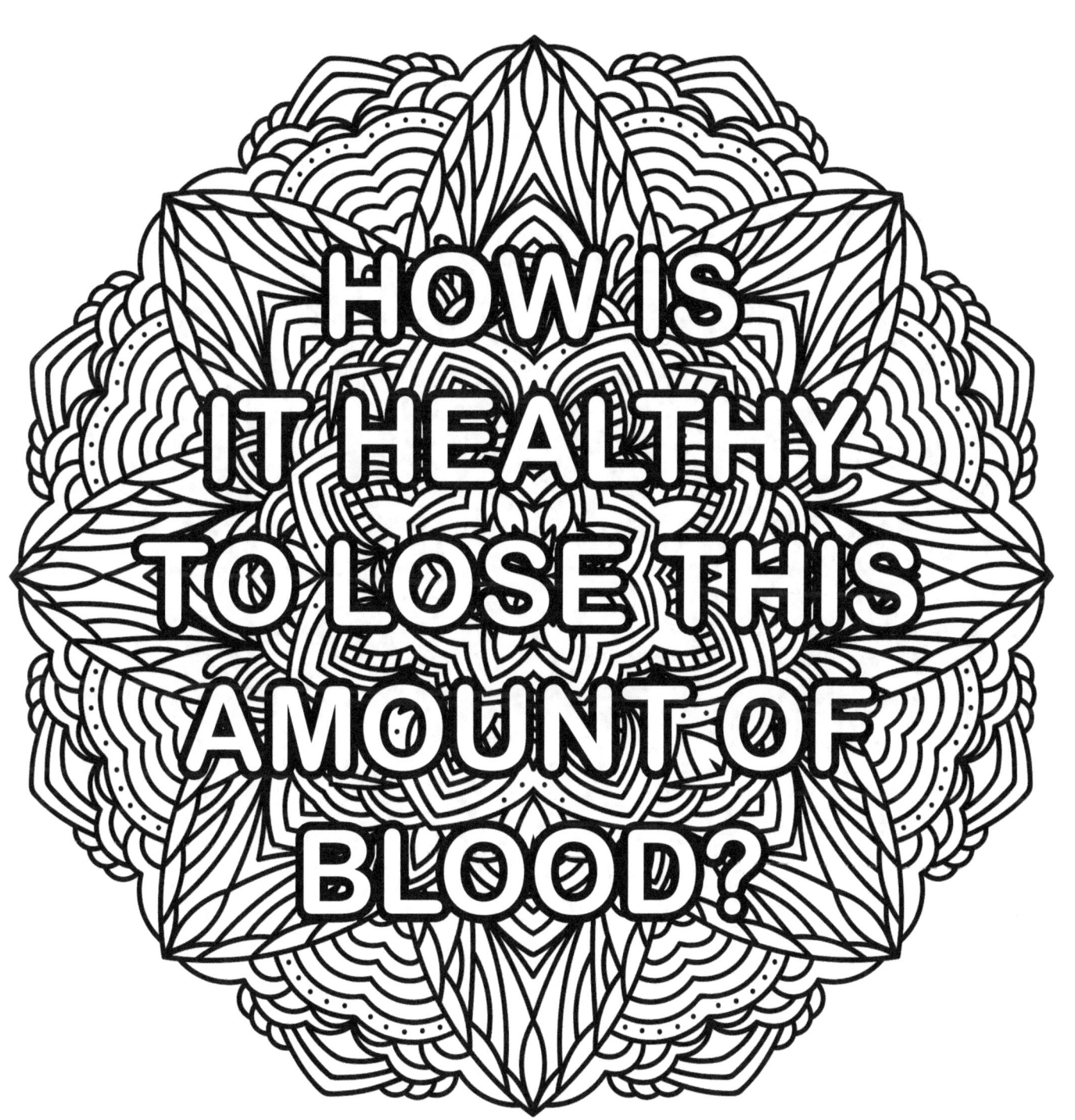

# COLORING CREW

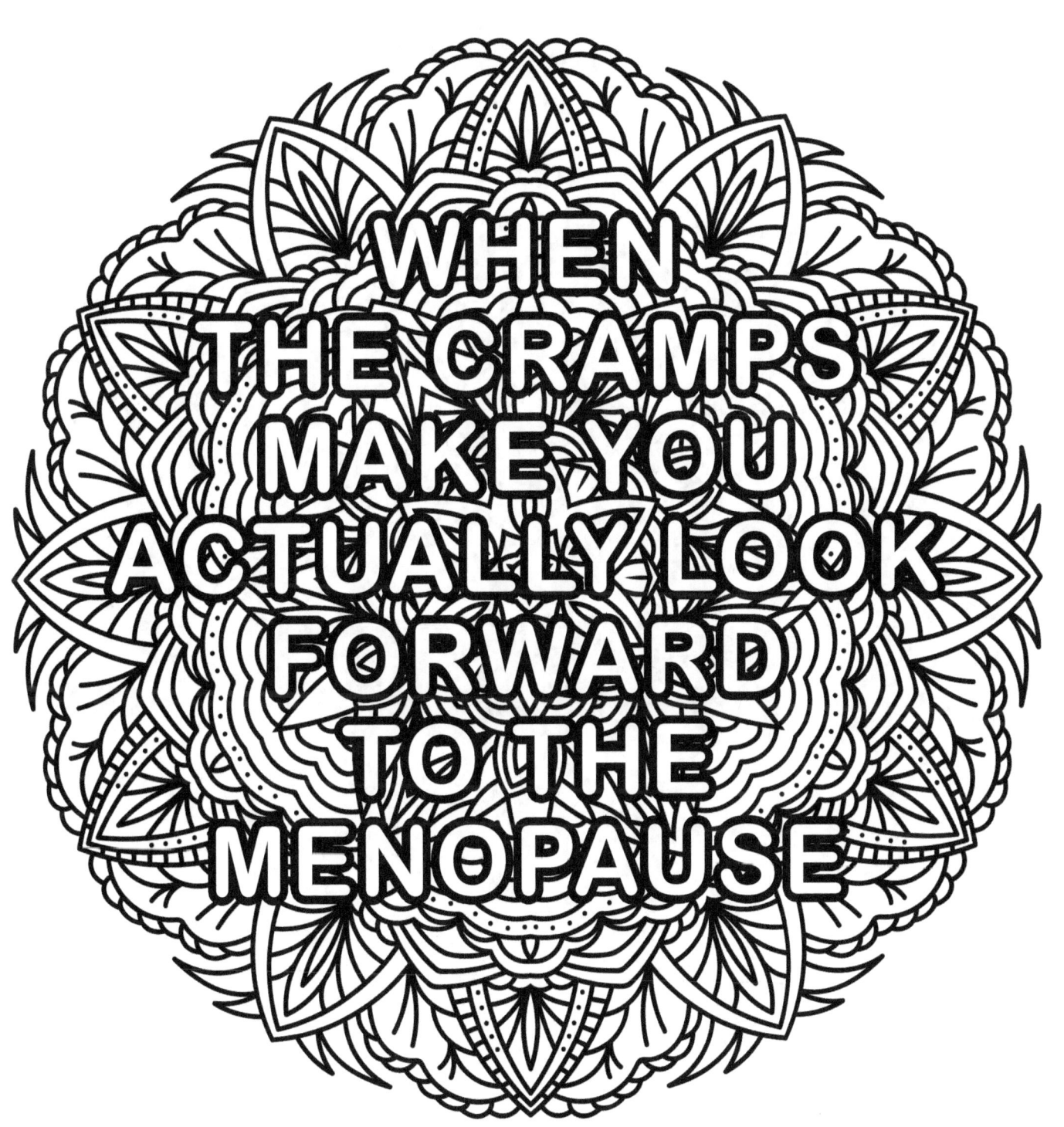

# COLORING CREW

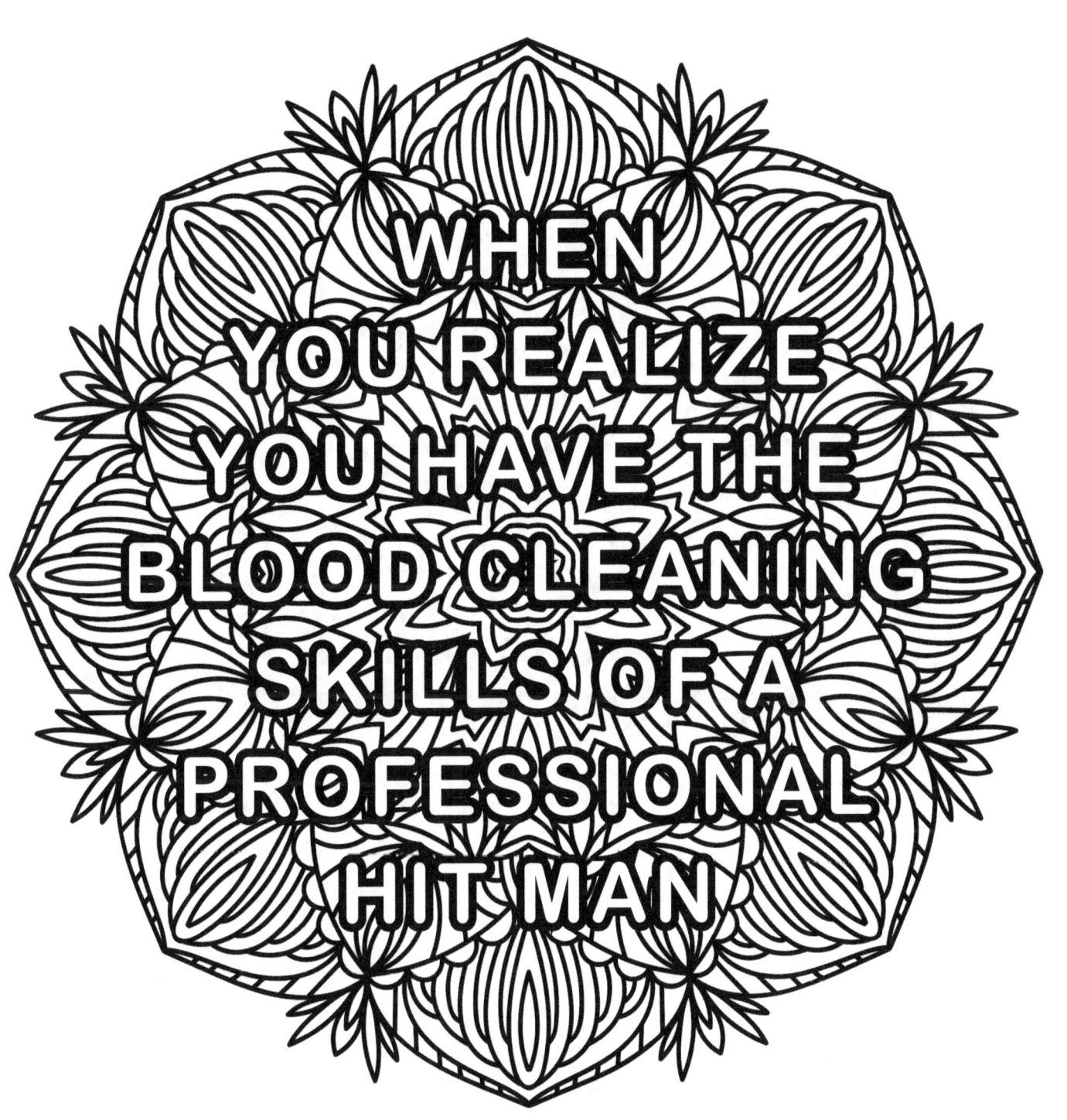

# COLORING CREW

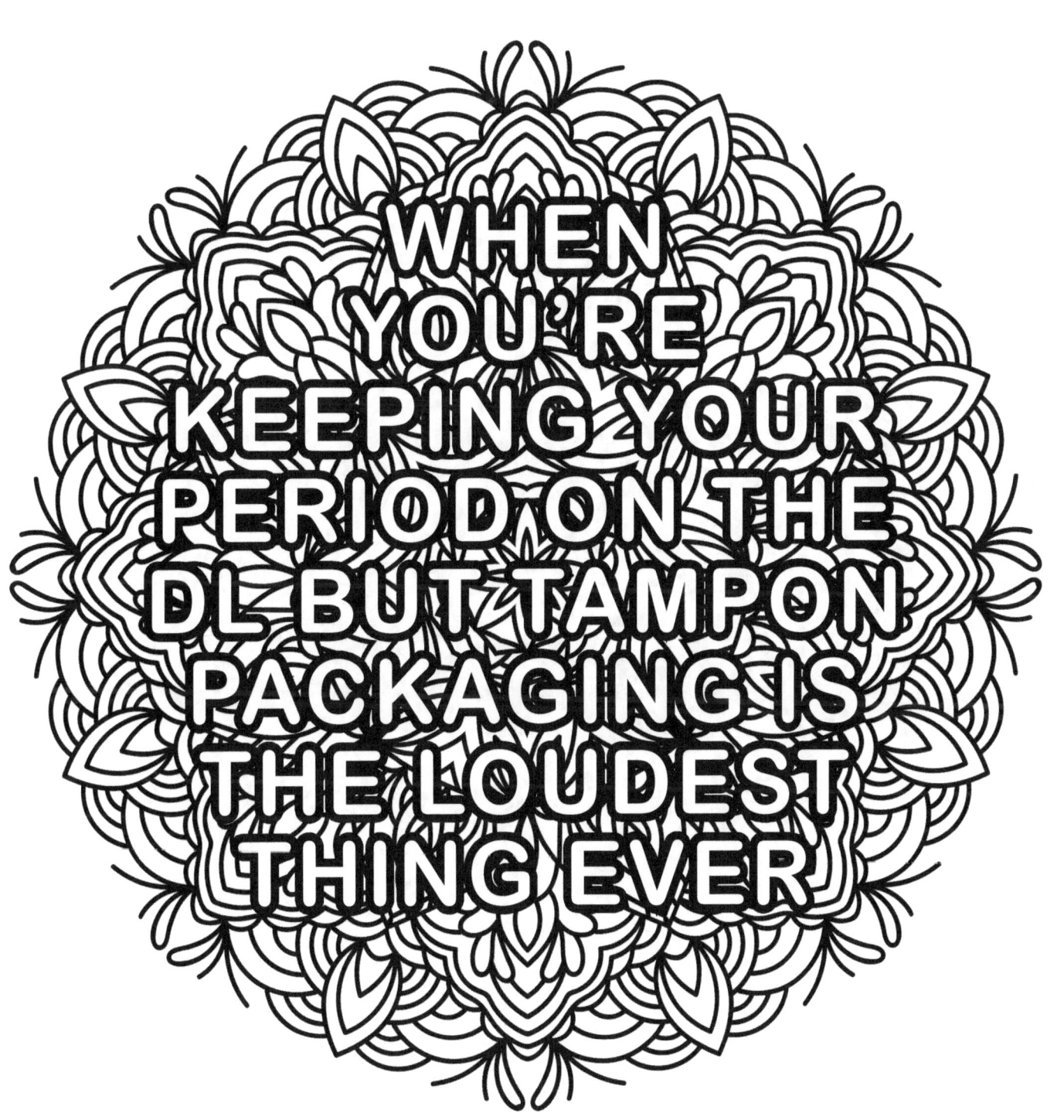

# COLORING CREW

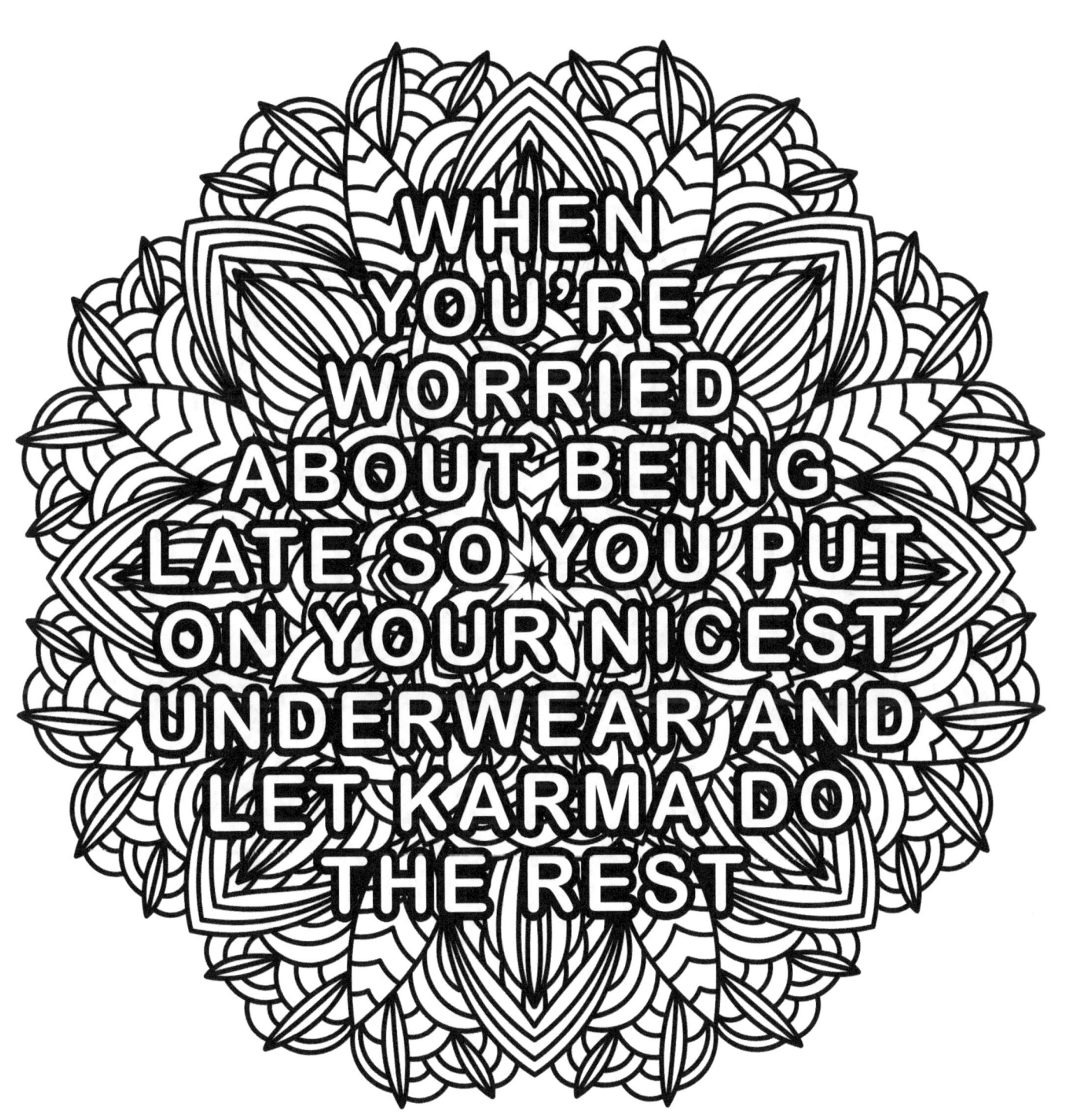

COLORING CREW

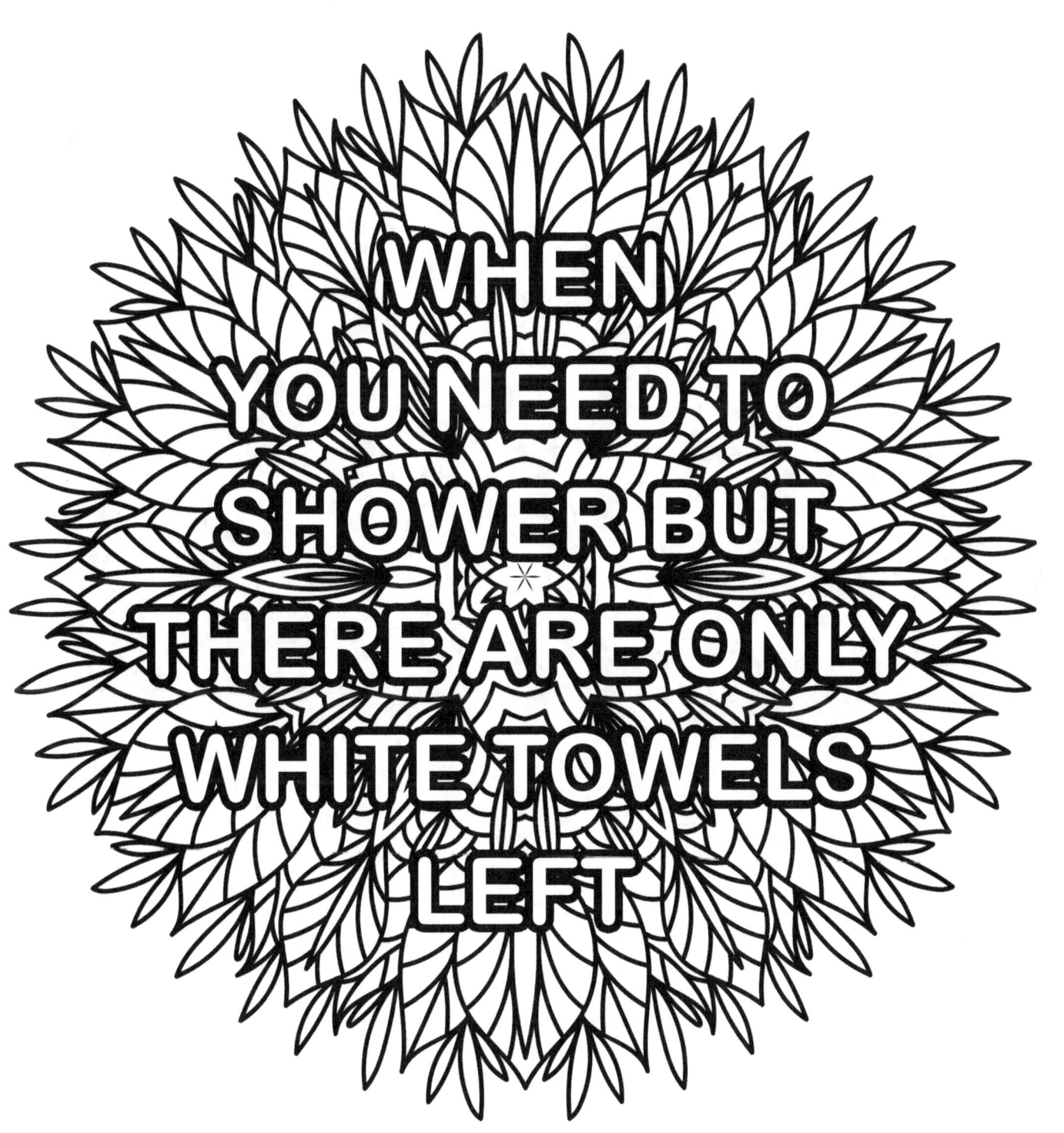

COLORING CREW

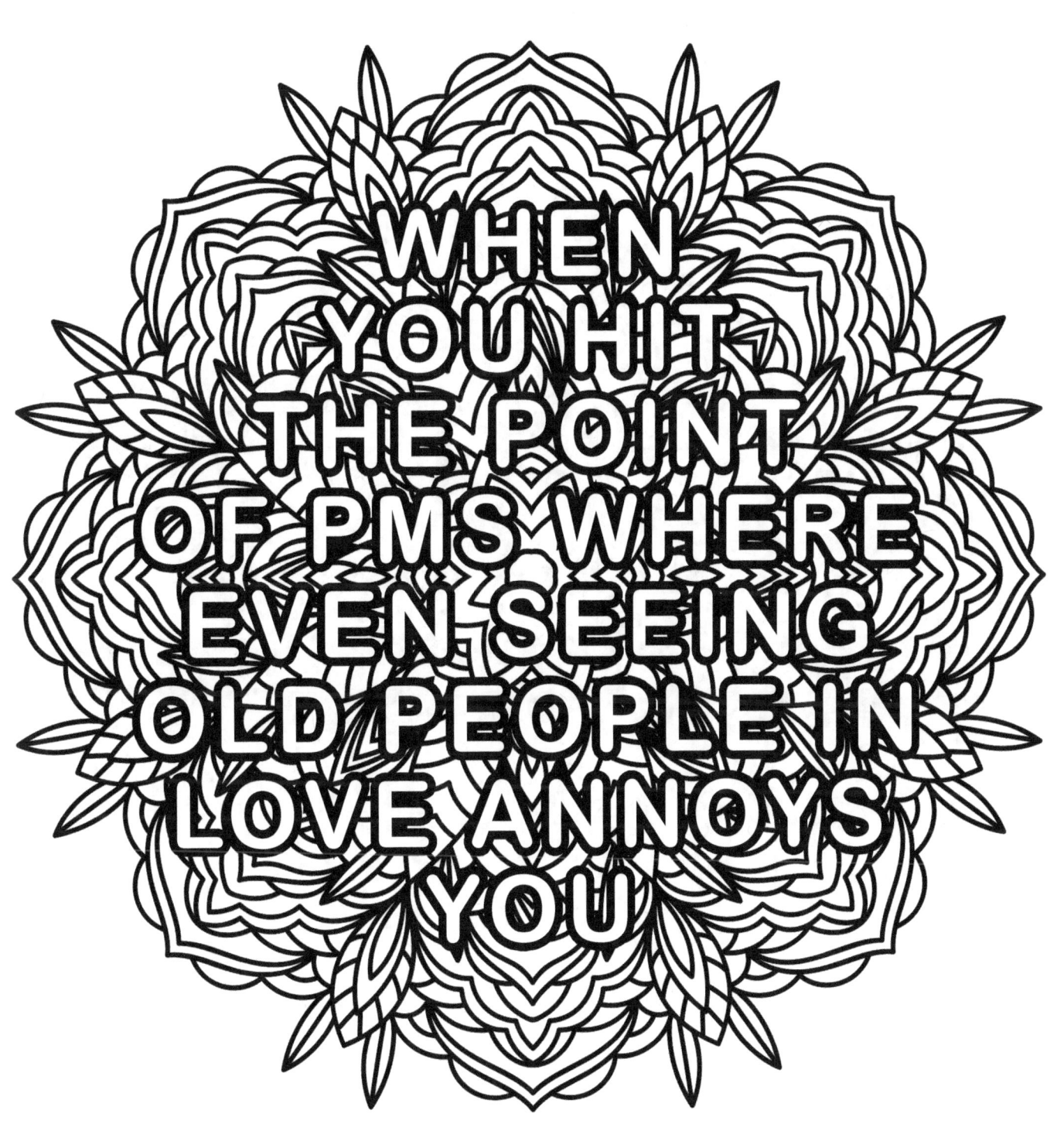

# COLORING CREW

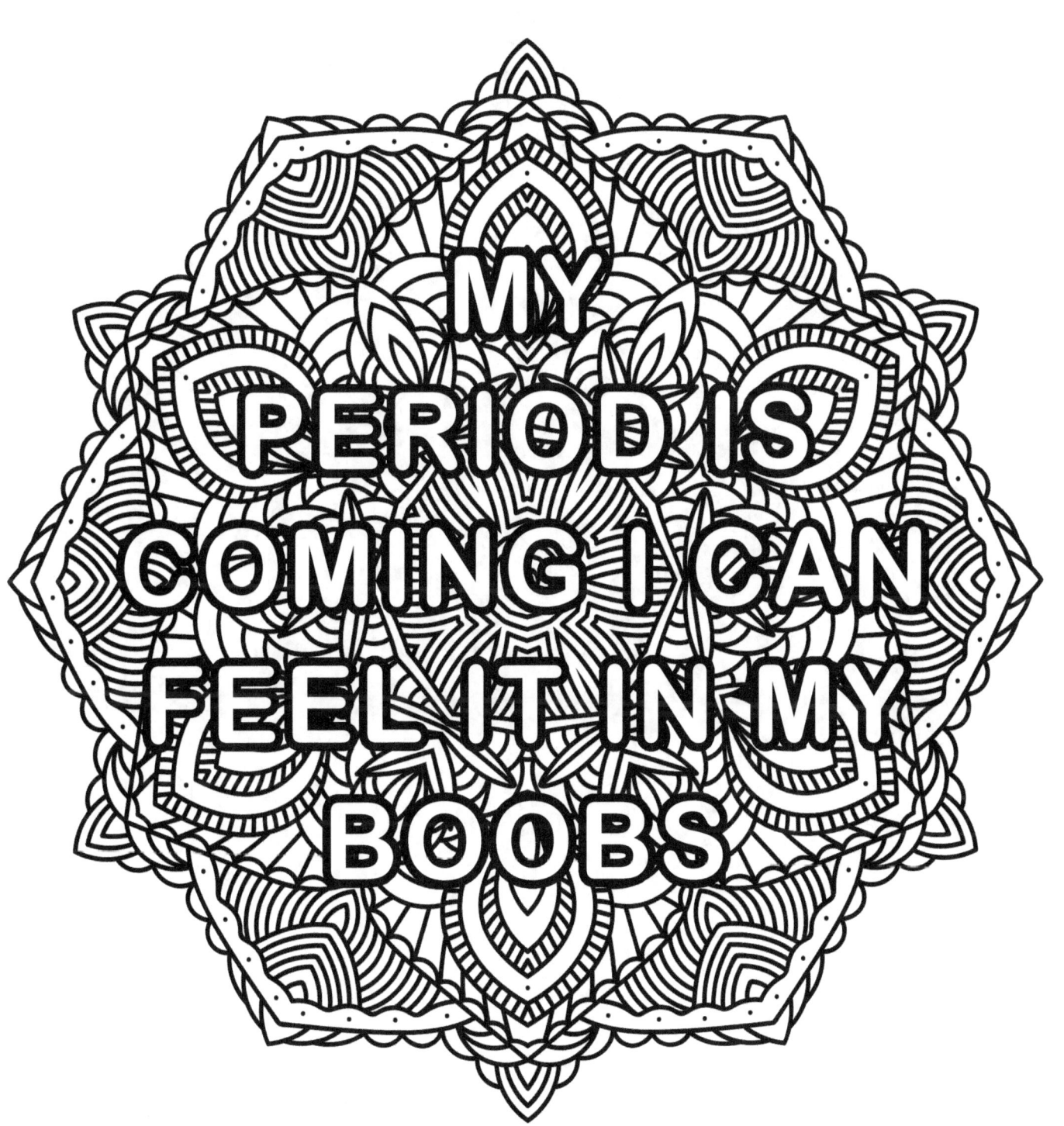

COLORING CREW

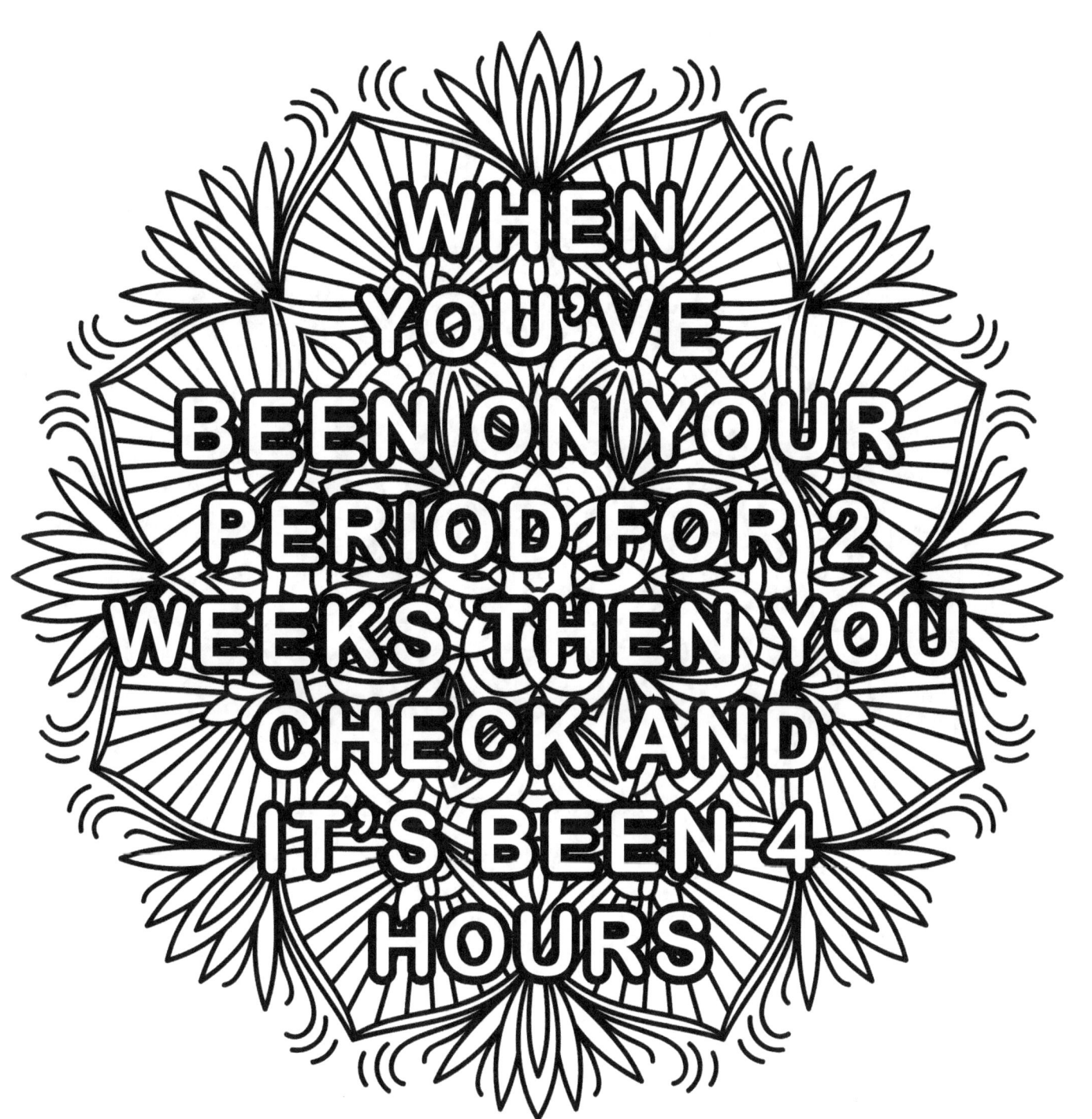

COLORING
CREW

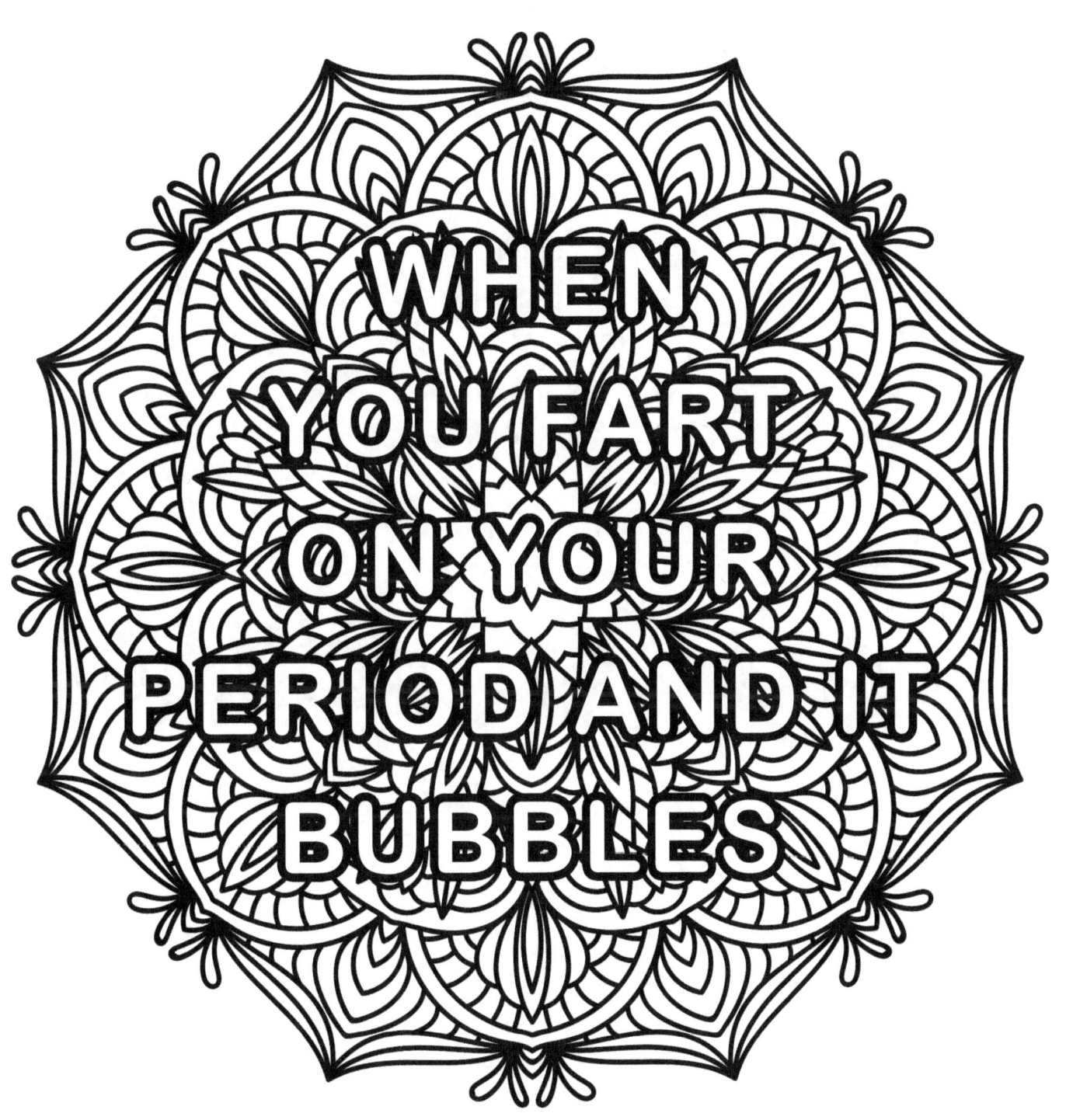

COLORING CREW

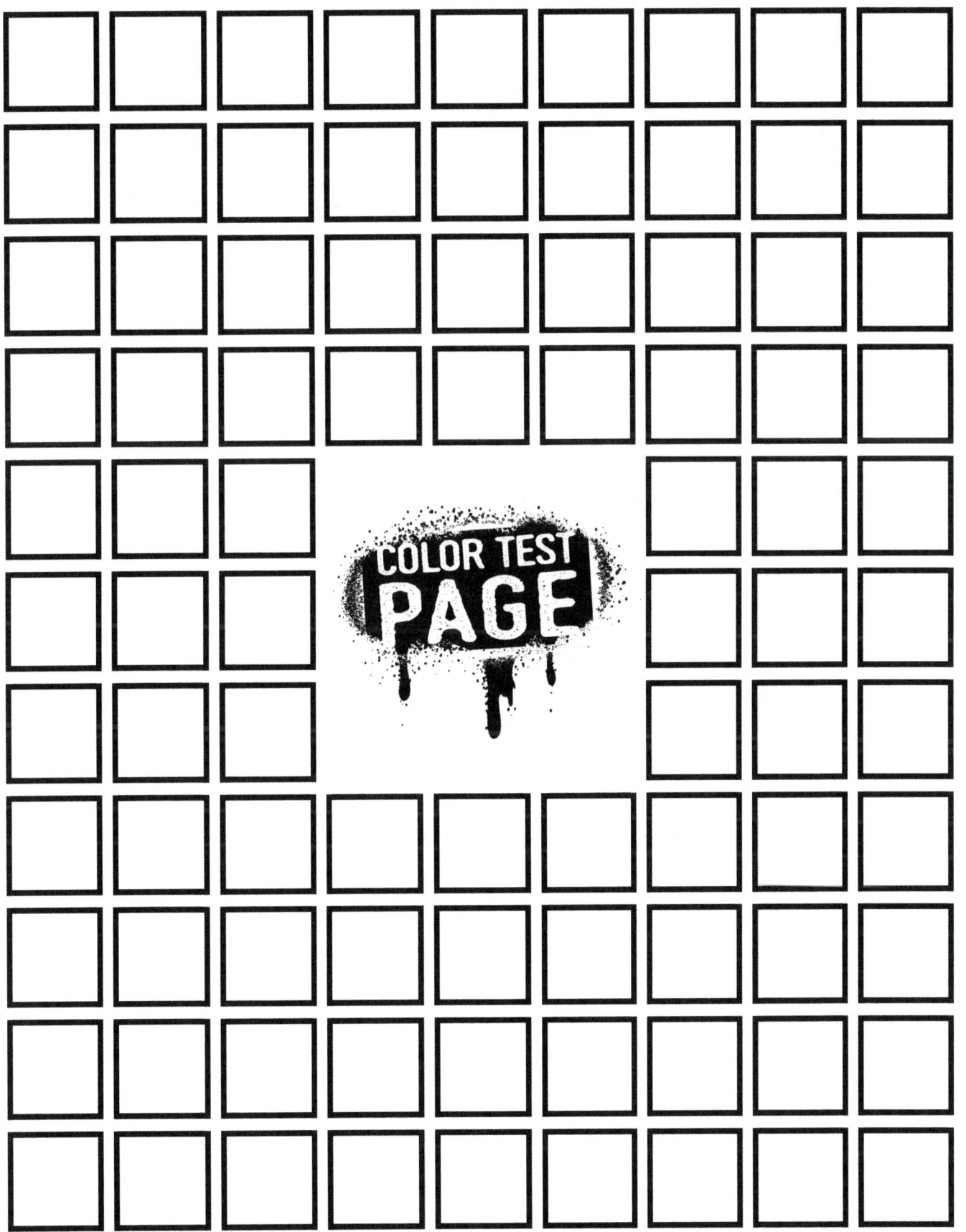

COLORING CREW

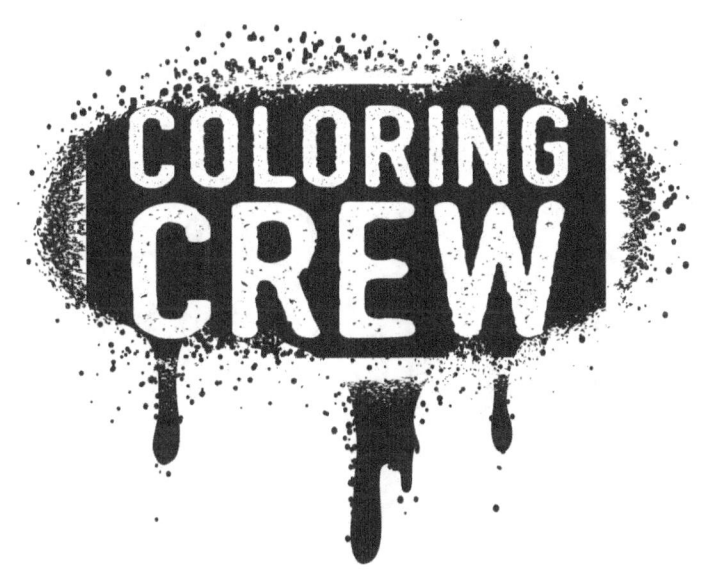

# THANKS!
# WE HOPE YOU HAD FUN!

IF YOU LIKED THIS BOOK THEN YOU YOU CAN VIEW OUR FULL RANGE OF HILARIOUS ADULT COLORING BOOKS BY GOING TO AMAZON AND SEARCHING FOR "COLORING CREW" AND THEN CLICKING ON OUR AUTHOR PAGE.

# THANKS AGAIN!

COLORING CREW

www.ingramcontent.com/pod-product-compliance
Lightning Source LLC
Chambersburg PA
CBHW062126220526
45471CB00010B/3896